Table of Contents

Unconventional Remedies for Clearing Congestion, Runny Nose, and Watery Eyes

Unconventional Allergy Symptom Relief Tips and Tricks

1. Introduction

Due to the profound impact allergies can have on quality of life and the uncertainty about when we will develop a solution, spending some time reviewing the potential value of some approaches that are either underexplored or have not been evaluated at all may be a good idea. We are considering treatments that need the least amount of clinician or therapist time, or that must be self-administered and will still be safe, even if they are ineffective. Though it is true that things that can boost the immune system or anti-inflammatory responses are worthwhile, there are other ways that allergy symptoms can be modified that have little to do with the actual system involved with allergies. This point is evidenced by the prevalence of the utilization of placebos in allergy research and the self-creation of placebo-like effects by the individual rumored to be "symptom-free" until eating a food they were avoiding due to allergy concerns. The subliminal placebo effect occurs when an individual is unaware that they are receiving a placebo and still report a reduction in symptoms.

Allergies occur when your immune system reacts to a foreign substance, such as a food item, medication, or pollen, that doesn't actually cause an issue for most people. Allergies are a common issue managed by doctors, but traditionally reducing contact with the allergenic substance, medications, or getting allergy shots or pills are used to mitigate the symptoms. This essay will discuss unconventional allergy symptom relief tips and tricks that may supplement such treatments, potentially avoiding medications or reducing the necessary dosage or side effect burden. Suggestions include taking a unique supplement or consuming a bit of local honey, proceeding with caution but potentially utilizing electroacupuncture, trying to change your thoughts and behavior, seeking out floatation REST techniques, and engaging in diaphragmatic breathing.

1.1. Understanding Allergies

Allergies occur with an exaggerated responsiveness of the body's immune defense system to certain environmental substances commonly referred to as allergens. Allergy symptoms are caused by substances in the air or food (allergens) to which a person is determined to be allergic. These symptoms arise when the allergen lands on the lining of the nose or the airways and leads to an allergic reaction. This allergic reaction manifests as irritation in the nose, sneezing, congestion, cold-like runny nose, or itching, as well as cough, chest congestion, wheezing, and shortness of breath. Some additional symptoms include itchiness of the mouth or throat, hives, itchy eyes, wheezing, and anxiety.

The most common top allergic triggers include animal allergy (dog, cat), dust mite allergy, insect sting allergy (bee, wasp, hornet, yellow jacket), mold allergy, pollen allergy (trees, grasses, and weeds), food allergy (milk, eggs, peanuts, wheat, soy, fish, shellfish), and latex allergy. The common symptoms of allergic reactions include itchiness, sniffles, hives, rashes, etc. Though these symptoms are considered common and temporary, in some selected cases and people, the exposure to their respective allergic triggers can result in serious health complications commonly known as anaphylaxis. Anaphylaxis results in emergency hospital treatment and can be life-threatening in some instances.

Allergies are one of the most common health issues experienced across the globe. In the United States alone, over 50 million people experience allergic reactions. Allergies occur when the body's immune response becomes hypersensitive to or has an exaggerated response to different environmental substances such as food, pollen, pet dander, mold, bee stings, etc. These different environmental substances, which are usually harmless, are called triggers or allergens.

2. Dietary Strategies

One idea is that the root of the allergy relief is the probiotics that are inside fermented foods. "Probiotics — the healthy bacteria in your gut — can have a lot to do with allergies," she says. To be more specific, several recent studies have found that probiotics can help prevent common allergies, like eczema, food allergies, and even seasonal allergies. In one study, toddlers who added fish oil and probiotics to their diet were up to 40% less likely to develop an allergy to milk than the placebos over a one-year period. In order to keep inflammation at bay, it's also a good idea to eat plenty of whole foods, like fruits and vegetables. Marie suggests the Mediterranean Diet to her patients with allergies or asthma, though not a large amount, because it features a huge amount of natural anti-inflammatories. You can think of the diet as an anti-inflammatory plan.

Experts assert that certain foods can make some allergy symptoms worse. Omega-3 fatty acids, for example, can serve as an anti-inflammatory agent, while the research on vitamin C shows that it may lower histamine levels, the compounds that catch a lot of the blame for uncomfortable symptoms. When it comes to fruits and veggies, the produce aisle is the place to go, experts say. Foods like oranges, broccoli, and bell peppers hold the important nutrient vitamin C – an antioxidant that may help keep the immune system in working order. Some scientists also believe that flavonoids, the compounds that give some fresh produce its bright colors, may help fight off free radicals and thus minimize allergy symptoms. Omega-3 foods like salmon, mackerel, and herring also have anti-inflammatory capabilities. One study found that kids who were exposed to the fruits and veggies had fewer allergies in general, which makes experts suspect that the mix of nutrients in the produce aisle can offer some level of decongestion.

2.1. Probiotics and Gut Health

Some of the trick to helping sustain healthy bacteria levels has to do with what your choices are: it turns out that healthy, whole food-based eating plans tend to support gut health and diversity. Here's where probiotics come in. The bacteria used in probiotics are similar types of bacteria that naturally live in your colon. By ingesting these "good" probiotic bacteria, the idea is that they can help replenish and level the playing field, putting yourself back in balance and thus promoting gut health. Much research considering how probiotics can help allergies are mostly small, and some conflicting results exist. Yet the bulk of people indicate potential, mainly for modulating the immune system in the gut. Since around 70% of your body's immune cells are located there, it makes sense that the immune response - or allergic response - in the gut can in turn impact the immune responses throughout the rest of your body. Probiotic use to temper allergic responses varies as well by the particular strain that's used, and, just like with eating foods to support your gut, more variety is usually thought to be more beneficial.

Alternative allergy relief opportunities don't just stop at essential oils! More research is starting to suggest that what's going on in your gut, in particular, might actually have an impact on your allergies. Specifically, some studies show a connection between the amount and diversity of bacteria in a person's gut and how their immune system responds to allergens. This could be particularly helpful for those with food allergies - rather than experiencing unexpected or alarming allergic symptoms, what if they could get a jump start on allergy relief by addressing their gut?

3. Lifestyle Adjustments

Reduced emphasis on control can leave symptom management feeling overwhelmingly difficult for those who struggle with it. By examining the mind's ebb and flow, interconnectedness, self-management and internal strength, self-therapy, arguably, may have a powerful effect. Our well-being and allergy symptoms might even be managed beyond typical physical and physiological medications, remedies and usage. Concentrating on lifestyle adjustments within the emotional, psychological, spiritual realm can make an equally, if not more, profound effect. Having an inspirational and caring healthcare professional can make all the difference, as their wisdom is invaluable and they provide unlimited support for you.

Exploring ways in which we might manage allergy symptoms, we can contemplate our mindsets, as well as our relationships to the world and those who share the environment with us. It goes without saying that stress can also trigger or exacerbate allergy symptoms. Mindfulness and stress management techniques could be equally as effective as antihistamines. Our autonomic nervous systems are programmed to heighten levels of alertness regarding potential threats to our well-being. Yet, through training, some are able to prime themselves to react differently, including to develop strategies surrounding mentalizations and resultantly, personal control and acumen. Reducing anxiety, stress and improving sleep quality tends to diminish allergic responses. Natural strategies like this can assist in reducing stress, which may lead to better management of allergy symptoms.

3.1. Mindfulness and Stress Management

In addition to mindfulness, the practice of ensuring that patients provoke red Ave in electrode without both trained and subjective immune effects does not change and penalize anxiety and fear. The amplification of the allergic relationship is the apex of travel, crossings, red wolves, and attacks on different systems of the rights food substance. It is also used to increase levels of adrenaline, reason, and cortisol. Normally, they are free to leave the psychoactive cortex of the hippocampus and cellulose and hope to become a Hutchison University unit for their knowledge and cause autism. The quality of secretion looks like a car compound up to the adult allowance is a basis due to cortisol's scaring and sicknesses and libido. In the last sample of all that is involved, Hiropon, the breathing also helps protect your body and psychological health to relieve stress and power, a powerful symptom reducer.

Another important gig with regard to mental health and allergies is a mindful attitude, oscillation, and stress management. Adhesive and Jansen provide many examples based on a literature review indicating a significant positive relationship between depression symptoms, increased allergies, and leading levels of positive emotions. Although there are few studies on the influence of mindfulness on allergy management, trauma and stress management are useful in reducing stress and anxiety, while also avoiding stress-related allergies. Mainstream-based cognitive therapy, which includes various components of healing, essence, and healing, has shown potential for a special all-pat index. Ideas that precede and develop for the way of life today can help improve allergies and the whole process.

4. Environmental Modifications

There are many different types of air purifiers and filters out there on the market, and those with allergies often seek allergy symptom relief by purchasing one for their homes. But do effective air purifiers make a difference when it comes to relieving allergy symptoms? The truth is that machines described as "air purifiers" do not reduce symptoms for all types of allergies. Depending on the type of air purifier you are thinking of getting, airborne particles may still make their way to the respiratory system in your body. Rooms are also structured in such a way that particles can continue to flow throughout them after coming into contact with the surfaces of those rooms. For these reasons, make sure to investigate both products and even whole-home systems that can also include filtered air into heater units.

One of the most tried and true methods for obtaining relief from allergy symptoms is to take steps to modify the environment in which allergy sufferers spend time. Pollen and dust are two of the most common triggers for allergies. Simply taking steps to avoid coming in contact with allergy triggers can go a long way toward relieving symptoms. People who have pet allergies might find relief from their symptoms if they visit people's houses that are free from pets, and people who react to pollen may find their symptoms are better in indoor, sealed-up homes with the air conditioning/heating on during high-pollinating seasons. An additional method of environmental modification is knowing self-avoidance techniques, or ways to stay away from particles that trigger your immune system, and preventing such materials from being tracked throughout buildings.

4.1. Air Purifiers and Filters

Air purifiers and filters have been shown to reduce the levels of dust mites and molds in the home, factors directly related to allergic conditions like asthma. Hospital-grade air purifiers, namely those with HEPA filters and ultraviolet lights, are considered by some as the future for mold control in homes. These systems have been shown to kill or inactivate 99.9 percent of mold spores and can trap 90 percent of the larger dust particles. The less the immune system has to deal with, the better. Another factor to consider is that since most of us spend the majority of our lives indoors, poor indoor air quality can have a serious effect on a sufferer of respiratory ailments such as allergies and asthma. Some of them are portable and some require professional installation.

Sometimes, in the pursuit of unconventional allergy treatments, it is easy to overlook interventions that actually address the outdoor threats unrelated to food and chemicals. Many allergy sufferers are advised to stay indoors on days with excessive pollen or when the air pollution is too high. Those who cannot or refuse to stay indoors are given more conventional advice. But the reasoning is sound. At its core, anyone interested in naturally managing their allergies needs to be taken out of the polluted air now and then. However, it does not have to be either outside living with the allergens or indoors cleaning with chemicals. Two "alternative" treatments for allergies focus on purifying the air within the home.

5. Alternative Therapies

Acupressure and acupuncture have been well-documented in studies to be useful in managing allergy symptoms. Acupressure relies on applying pressure to the same points used in acupuncture to relieve various types of pain and discomfort with an application of pressure. Acupuncture uses small and very thin needles to unblock "chi" or "life force" and is thought to correct imbalances in the body that cause discomfort and, in the case of allergies, sinus pain and pressure. Both practices have been lauded as a great supplement or alternative to oral medications and prescription drugs in alleviating ongoing symptoms.

Alternative therapies may be helpful for some people. Always check with a doctor before beginning an alternative therapy. Below are some examples of non-medication allergies and their level of evidence supporting their use. Allergies are one example of the use of acupuncture to relieve symptoms. A good place to start researching alternative therapies is to look at patient blogs or healthcare articles on the internet that discuss why therapies work. Find out what works for people and have tried and tested methods of relief on your body. Keep in mind that results are not always consistent for individuals, and alternative therapies are not as widely studied as other medicines.

Many individuals suffering from seasonal allergies have found relief from their symptoms using alternative therapies. Alternative therapies are considered medical interventions that aren't taught widely in medical schools, aren't used in our hospitals, and are not generally considered a first line of treatment. But for those suffering from allergies, antihistamines and prescription medications often prescribed to relieve symptoms are not enough. For individuals with life-threatening allergies, our doctors recommend traditional medical practice.

5.1. Acupuncture and Acupressure

In Traditional Chinese Medicine, acupuncture and acupressure are founded on the concept of "Qi," which is the flow of energy within the body. It is believed that when a person experiences allergies, they have bodily blockages. Acupressure ensures energies are aligned by balancing the yin and yang, which are believed to account for immune function. By equilibrating these energies, the body can fight off the intrusion of allergens. Additionally, acupressure aids the release of histamine, the root of allergy symptoms. Studies suggest that acupressure can help to alleviate hives. William Osler, a 19th-century Canadian physician, is thought to have driven the introduction of acupuncture in the Western world for issues such as allergies, though evidence based around allergies and acupuncture remains fairly sparse. Furthermore, little is known about how and why acupuncture and acupressure work in the context of allergies, but many have found them beneficial. Acupuncture involves needles inserted in the skin, so those who have a fear of needles might feel better using acupressure.

Many individuals experience allergies in one form or another, and the typical path for relief involves medication or the use of air filters. What if you wanted to try a less invasive approach for allergy-related relief? This is not to discredit traditional methods as they are effective. Nonetheless, there are some who want to try alternative therapies. Acupuncture and acupressure may be a good bet for allergy control. They've been around for over 3,000 years and have been shown to be effective for a wide array of issues, including allergies. China has utilized both techniques for tens of centuries, and both were introduced to Westerners as a result of a Swedish missionary's voyage through China. Since then, acupressure and acupuncture have grown popular in some Western countries as alternative therapies for allergies and other conditions.

6. Herbal Remedies and Supplements

Quercetin supplements are typically taken in doses from 500 to 1000 milligrams three times daily. The supplement form of quercetin seems to work the best for allergies used in people suffering from hay fever. When far more food is used that provides quercetin, natural supplements are for improving athletic performance. Some may also develop a rash after taking it. It may be taken as a syrup, tincture, or tea in powdered or capsule form. Herbalists may prescribe hawthorn to improve the cardiovascular system and help mitigate symptoms of asthma and hay fever. Scientists believe there is a connection between heart health and hay fever, as both have causes linked to inflammation.

Intriguingly enough, a lot of allergy sufferers also turned to natural remedies for relief, ranging from honey and apple cider vinegar to herbal remedies and dietary supplements. Some of the most common include butterbur, which functions as an antihistamine, and works best when taken regularly at least two weeks before allergies bother you. Butterbur's active ingredient is petasin. It is advised not to take butterbur supplements due to the risk of liver damage; instead, extract forms are recommended as they remove harmful plant chemicals. Sometimes, butterbur may cause belching, diarrhea, difficulty breathing, fatigue, headache, hives, itching, red eyes, discoloration and swelling of the skin, or stomach upset. It may counteract complications during pregnancy and breastfeeding. Another recommended herbal remedy is quercetin, a flavonoid that reduces mast cells in the airways' release of histamine. It is found in tea, red wine, Akar, citrus fruits, and onions, as well as in supplement form.

6.1. Butterbur and Quercetin

A bioflavonoid like resveratrol, quercetin contributes to plants' pigmentation and provides anti-histamine and anti-inflammatory properties. Quercetin is also known to help clear up certain allergic signs and symptoms like nasal congestion, itchy and watery eyes, sneezing, and hives. To this day, studies of quercetin's capability regarding treating allergic reactions in humans have been fairly minimal. Moreover, our body does not absorb quercetin nearly as well. To enhance quercetin's absorption, some health professionals propose coupling the supplement with an enzyme known as bromelain.

Cultures around the world have long been using these herbs as historical medicines. Butterbur is a plant native to a number of areas situated in the northern hemisphere. The plant boasts anti-inflammatory as well as antihistaminic properties. The two components in butterbur that produce these effects are isopetasin and petasin. If you want to make use of this herb, though, doctors generally suggest finding a butterbur supplement that has undergone some sort of safe extraction that gets rid of these herbs' toxic elements.

7. Innovative Technologies

Consider using apps that track, but remember that it's important to connect with your healthcare provider to track trends or concerns in symptoms. Pharmacists may act as an advisor to inform healthcare providers about medications and pharmacy waits, not diagnosing or treating you. It should also be noted that telephone offer tracking receptors to those using their medications. So, as a general rule, be skeptical of claims made by some of the technological tools available to us through smartphones. When it comes to health, effective and safe allergy symptom tracking management typically involves the regular supervision of your healthcare professional.

As technology progresses, we find that the management of allergies deepens with the integration of various advanced tools and technologies. A quick search in the App Store or Google Play for "allergy," "food allergy," or "medication tracking" will yield proven and unproven smartphone apps to assist in managing your symptoms. Apps that pertain to allergies include simply tracking and management symptoms. Others may include recipes, ways to manage food at restaurants, information on multiple allergens, such as food, medication and latex, and much more. Most of the apps were developed by consumers, so if the development of tracking allergies seems to be taking a long time, or if an existing app doesn't have all the features needed, there are templates and programming to develop your own application.

7.1. Smartphone Apps for Allergy Tracking

Arun B. Patel, PharmD, an assistant professor of pharmacy at the University of Pittsburgh, advises the individuals he works with to download MyHives, an app developed by Allergy & Asthma Network. With this app, patients are able to select the affected area on a human graphic, along with severity, on a 0-10 point scale. Patel contends patients utilizing the app are more likely to return with relevant data. "It has been a way for me to improve my history taking," he reports. "Picture continuation can be really helpful." Allergy Link, developed by Children's Hospital of Colorado, is another user-friendly app designed to help identify specific allergens or irritants that might be causing someone's symptoms by connecting them to an individual in the allergy department at the children's hospital in Colorado by a video interface. Developed by a pharmaceutical company, the restoration version of the app is called MyEpiPen, which lists the medications that have been prescribed to and gives users some basic guidance. Further reading through the app is available for users. Management of allergy can be effectively accomplished through highlighting QR codes on new Apfel CBD allergy labels to give users a comprehensive understanding of where specific allergies are originated from.

With advancements in modern technology, more people turn to their smartphones for help in managing their health. One app, Zyrtec AllergyCast, offers hex color codes to describe the day's pollen count and forecast. Other allergy apps can create logs of your antihistamine usage, set up dosing reminders, and even include a list of allergist-recommended cleaning products. Rather than sticking to just one for your daily tracking, these apps can be utilized in conjunction to actively monitor your allergies. Keeping track of both OTC and prescription meds will give a more comprehensive view of successful treatments. Smartphone apps are compatible with both iOS and Android operating systems.

8. Uncommon Practices

Many holistic wellness practices include the use of a "salt cave," also known as "halotherapy." Salt caves are constructed utilizing the same surfaces that are used to establish a saltwater fish tank. As individuals breathe in the salty air, it can help to reestablish a neutral pH in the body, open airways, ease irritation from swollen adenoids and tonsils in kids, and even cure skin conditions. According to Ben Reuter, owner of Breathe Salt Vault, the negative ions in the salt can help individuals breathe better, relieve anxiety, avoid sinus infections, and even exterminate virus in the air. Reuter explains that although some people might visit the salt cave a couple of times a week, everyone is unique, and a little might go a long way—not to mention being costly. A common recommendation is to use it in conjunction with routine daily allergy treatments and, of course, to speak with a doctor for other unrelated health issues. Always consult your doctor.

Consider the possibility that there are some unusual practices that are highly effective at helping relieve allergy symptoms. As strange as it may seem, some people report feeling better in some environments. These tips are, unfortunately, not supported by scientific studies. Your doctor is the source of real knowledge, and he or she should be consulted. The list below is presented in no particular order. When you enter a new environment, it is

imperative that you keep an open and curious attitude.
Have fun.

8.1. Halotherapy and Salt Caves

A 2016 paper reviewed the possible anti-inflammatory actions of inhaled hypertonic saline. According to background written by the doctors, cystic fibrosis patients are treated with inhalable saltwater to help clear their airways. One systematic review of studies suggested this could also be helpful for controlling the symptoms of severe asthma, which could be related to allergic reactions. Whether inhaled salt (like that used in cystic fibrosis studies) helps is considered less of a chance by the researchers because of the higher concentration used. But for that matter, the data is weak for this therapy at all and more research is needed to be sure. The idea is that because salt can absorb water, it causes the mucus lining the airway to dry out and that might help allergies in a different way.

In the heart of Poland, in the town of Wieliczka, there is a salt mine that has been operational since medieval times and is now a famous tourist spot. Opened in 2012, it offers something called the Kinga Spa, with an underground salt lake and floating therapy. There are salt caves throughout the area where one can receive an underground mani-pedi or facial. Salt is also getting attention as a treatment for nasal symptoms. While it cannot replace traditional allergy medications like antihistamines, it may be helpful for some. The idea of breathing in salt therapy, or halotherapy, isn't new and has seen a resurgence in recent years.

9. Combination Approaches

Interpersonal psychotherapy is a psychotherapy that works toward focusing on the relationships an individual has with others or indeed themselves. An analysis published in the British Medical Journal reports that non-adherence with guideline treatment for allergic rhinitis actually is related to depression rather than the severity of an individual's symptoms. Therefore, take the time to explore herbs such as butterbur, essential oils like peppermint, and incorporating environments that have music therapy into your life.

When in doubt, talk with your provider or allergist about a plan for managing your symptoms. They should be able to guide you in the right direction and monitor your health as well. Set goals, and include some measures of improvement. For example, track the number of times you require your rescue inhaler. If you have an EpiPen and suffer from food allergies, discuss whether using it at the same time as another sort of allergy medication can help avoid the symptoms or progression of anaphylactic allergy symptoms.

It is possible and indeed may be more effective to take a combination approach to dealing with allergies. Consider taking some time to develop a personalized protocol to manage your symptoms this season. For example, combining the activity of yoga with deep breathing exercises can improve long-term quality of life among those dealing with allergic reactions. Some studies suggest that a more clinical approach of combining drugs known as bronchodilators and antileukotrienes is effective among individuals with asthma. There are also several studies reporting that combined sublingual or subcutaneous allergen immunotherapy and omalizumab elicits desensitization to food or inhaled allergens. In other words, using both in tandem can reduce symptoms, improve quality of life, and lead to profound changes in quality of life.

9. Combination Approaches

9.1. Yoga and Breathing Exercises

1.2. Breathing Exercises – Breathing exercises are some of the most effective ways to relieve both mental and physical tensions. By combining essential oils with these, a person can help release endorphins and other neurotransmitters, improve immune response, and buffer stress or anxiety. Inhaling eucalyptus oil or diffusing it during the practice of these exercises can stimulate the respiratory tracts to aid in inspiration and exhalation, clearing up sinus issues. When practicing these breathing exercises, position your body in a comfortable seat and take long, deep breaths with your mouth open. Place a damp cloth or some eucalyptus oil in the nose, bringing the air through the mouth and out the nasal passageways. Breathe in slowly and hold it for a couple of seconds, then release it slowly through your nostrils. This exercise helps increase lung capacity and improve overall lung function while reducing anxiety. It's also great for opening up the nasal passages and relieving allergy symptoms.

1.1. Try Yoga – Yoga is a wonderful way for people to relieve stress. The poses combine gentle movements with deep breathing exercises. These exercises use a form of breathing that not only relaxes the person but also allows for more oxygen to be taken in. This is beneficial for muscle relaxation and reducing allergic responses.

While allergies are nothing to sneeze at, there are methods that you can use for effective allergy symptom relief. The goal is to use a natural approach that has a proven track record of helping people feel better. This section can go over some of those methods in brief, highlighting how they can practice these techniques for immediate benefit. These include:

10. Conclusion

Adaptability and a willingness to try new things are a major part of life for those suffering from an allergy. A lack of understanding seems to go hand-in-hand with allergies, never playing by the rules or giving a cast-iron promise that good days are just around the corner. This lack of general awareness about the realities of life with allergies can make things even harder, resulting in some sufferers feeling incredibly alienated. To try and manage some of these feelings, as well as managing the symptoms themselves, processes are often relied on to create a sense of calm and assurance. This essay shows the importance of hearing a range of voices and diversity in approaches for establishing relief from allergy symptoms.

In conclusion, we find that this essay has explored the broad topic of unconventional allergy tips and has outlined 10 ideas to assist allergy sufferers in avoiding some of the worst seasonal symptoms. The individuals featured in this essay used a variety of digital communication styles, such as blog posts, videos, podcast transcripts, and a guest post on a journal blog, and offered their advice in prose as well as through images. The final essay is presented as a slideshow video presentation, which provides a harmonizing visual element to unite the diverse range of media and is also available as a document transcript for accessibility. This essay successfully highlights a range of strategies sought out by allergy sufferers to alleviate their symptoms.

Some hints offer dietary and lifestyle changes that can alleviate the discomfort of allergies. The use of ginger, onions, and garlic in cooking, living in mountains with increased air quality, driving with the car windows down due to high pollen concentration, and the use of fragrance-free personal hygiene products and fluoride-free or distilled water are examples of these recommendations. Fly traps, air purifiers, and mattress, window, and vacuum cleaners may also be useful in allergy relief. A range of ear wax-removal methods, bowel movement, masturbation, oregano oil, and so on may have casual suggestions that are less supportive.

Meditation, mindfulness, deep breathing, heated lamps, and saunas, and reduced sugar intake have been revealed by some scientific evidence to reduce the effects of allergies. New research also shows that children given antibiotics have a higher risk of developing allergies later in life because the chemicals change the bacterial balance in the stomach, leading to differences in immune system function. Regular cleaning can also make an important impact on allergy symptoms, as allergen accumulations can occur on places like airplane seats or even in the office at work. A probiotic could also be taken, as they can help establish a healthier stomach balance and also decrease the risk of developing eczema.

Recognizing that conventional allergy medications simply aren't effective for all allergy sufferers is important. For example, it may be helpful to pair conventional medications with natural remedies. Caffeine is available over the course of the day, and moderate amounts of caffeine can increase the effectiveness of certain decongestant medications. Showering allergens prior to bed can keep pollen and spores out of the bed. A saline wash is also useful, as it can sometimes prevent the use of steroids and other decongestants. If a saline wash is unavailable, a wash with a diluted mild hypoallergenic detergent can also be effective.

While traditional cold remedies are often loaded with carbohydrates, a new natural remedy is recommended, which involves consuming a tea made of honey, cinnamon, turmeric, a couple slices of fresh ginger, black pepper, and lemon. A variety of herbal teas as well as mint and sage candies can be helpful for asthma. Inhaling eucalyptus and peppermint oil can also serve as a decongestant for the airways. Although proper hydration is always recommended, as well as adequate vitamin intake, these practices may be even more useful during allergy season. Research has also shown that local honey may be a useful preventative for allergies to local pollinating plants.

Blot the nose and avoid blowing it, while not as effective, to reduce re-irritation from the nose due to constant blowing. Steam inhalation can be used to alleviate nasal and chest congestion, where the individual should inhale steam from a hot running shower. To soothe a sore throat, saltwater gargling and throat lozenges can coat the throat, the former of which can kill bacteria if used in the form of saltwater. Clear sinuses can be achieved through a natural saline nasal spray, used frequently to help encourage mucus drainage.

For those who suffer from eye irritations, the use of moist heat relief can be soothing and reduce redness and eye irritation. Another eyewash solution includes a saline sodium solution in which the individual should lean their head backwards and roll their eyeballs around, exposing the entire eye to the solution.

Allergies can wreak havoc with their symptoms. While many people use pharmaceuticals and over-the-counter medications to address allergy symptoms, it may benefit some individuals to consider alternative and/or adjunct therapies. These suggestions are believed to help people find relief from various allergy symptoms.

Unconventional Remedies for Clearing Congestion, Runny Nose, and Watery Eyes

1. Introduction

In conclusion, this essay is dedicated to discussing some non-traditional treatments to help clear the nose to the point that congestion no longer clogs up the passages, so that the nose can be so clear that it does not drip or run anymore. As a possible result of the alleviation of congestion, some other problems may also be lessened as well. A runny nose should not be stopped if it is needed for cleaning the nose, but why should it need to drip or run if the nose has been cleared of its congestion. So, to make a distinction, non-traditional ways to not stop a runny nose, and to not cause a runny nose, are being addressed in this essay.

A runny nose indicates that, although there are signs of a healthy, permeable nose, the nose becomes clogged from time to time so that it drips or runs. The drainage that is seen as a runny nose is often a form of the nose dripping its cleansing solutions if the nose were allowed to remain in its healthy, declogged state. If the nose were clogged up as this cleansing solution were to be secreted in the nose, the extremes of runny nose or stuffy nose might not occur.

Though decongestants, antihistamines, and surgeries have great impacts on clearing congestion, drying up the runny nose, and drying up watery eyes, these options are not realistic forms of treatment for people to use to stop congestion, a runny nose, and watery, itchy eyes in a natural way. When decongestants dry up the nose, they do so in a way that is not natural and forces people to breathe more through their mouths than through their noses. Decongestants may have the same net effect of decongestion amount as these natural, non-traditional treatments that are listed below, but they do so in a forced, unnatural manner.

1.1. Background and Significance

Often, conventional therapies for several allergy symptoms are not very effective or, if they are, treatment is usually for a very short medication trial. Some treatments may result in side effects that make the medication not worth taking. For example, side effects of antihistamines and decongestants used for symptoms of rhinitis may include too much drying causing nosebleeds or too dry a mouth; an endocrine dyscrasia with too little estrogen and too much testosterone leading to lip syndrome; prostate problems with dribbling or urinary symptoms; or drowsiness in the elderly, which can result in falls. In persons with dry AMD, decongestants and caffeine may exacerbate the problem. These are all reasons that some may choose not to use drugs at all, seek alternative medicine, or engage the care of a homeopath.

Many people have chronic allergies of several types that generally manifest as sneezing, congestion, runny nose, and watery eyes. These symptoms are usually worse upon awakening in the morning and again at bedtime. There are many conventional treatments for these symptoms, but they can also be a source of distress with many side effects, or they may not work for a particular individual. New ideas and drugs are needed. This manuscript will closely examine the evidence for unconventional treatments of a variety of sinus, nasal, and ocular symptoms, along with a discussion of what may be in the future of treatment options.

2. Congestion Relief Remedies

Cleavers was a traditional British remedy for cleansing the lymph system. The medicine is more easily made into a dense tea with chopped, fresh plant. The tea tastes fairly good; it is said to nourish dry mucous membranes, cleanses lymph and glandular system and detoxifies excess uric acid.

Warm, soothing foods such as broths, soup, and cooked grains are rich in enzymes as well as helpful to the body system for prevent gas, bloating, and stomach discomforts. If it is spicy food that will stimulate your immunity stress, stimulate your body power with spicy soup with spices such as turmeric, coriander seeds, and mustard seeds. Carrot-parsnip soup mixed with turmeric stimulate your liver bile and thus increases digestion secret and promotes liver friendliness.

If your nose is blocked, eat spicy food, hot chilies or peppers, horseradish, wasabi, and other hot peppers. Make sure to use thin-skinned, freshly frozen green chilies dropped in hot water and then chewed immediately. This could instigate release of mucus.

For a kid that has congestion, mix a child-spooning of honey, which is about 1/2 tablespoon, with six drops of tincture of black elderberry and give this by the kid's spoon three to five times a day. Another way to lessen congestion is to eat green onion, scallion, seaweed, and other members of the allium family, which include garlic.

Congestion could be remedied through present unconventional remedies. For congestion of the head, steam inhalation could be resorted to. Essential oils could be added to the water used for steam inhalation. Thyme, rosemary, and eucalyptus oil are antiseptic. Eucalyptus oil could produce a vapor that is good for healing the respiratory system.

2.1. Steam Inhalation with Essential Oils

In the traditional methods of steam inhalation, a few drops
of an essential oil are added to a pot of water. For folks
hoping to fight infections and clear sinuses, one might
choose from sage, rosemary, or eucalyptus. Adding one of
these essential oils will increase effectiveness towards
symptoms associated with head colds or infections. Some
other, sometimes more popular choices would be
chamomile or lavender. Both promote combinations of
calm and relief, something some people find very
appealing. "Lavender has been shown to decrease the
stress hormone cortisol" according to Meloni. Steam
inhalation can work for people in different ways and
choosing an essential oil that works best for the individual
is what is most important. Aromatherapist, Abigail Madden
adds that while inhaling steam, "Essential oils reach the
back of your nasal cavity and your sinus cavities, and also
40% of it is absorbed through your lungs." In addition to
curing whatever ails you, Madden explains, "It treats you
on an emotional level." Different oils can relieve anxiety,
stress, or depression and "all of these states can have an
impact on the physical body," says Madden.

One widely known and well-accepted practice for treating
a variety of ailments is the use of steam inhalation. Used
primarily for respiratory issues, particularly congestion,
steam inhalation is a simple remedy that calls for a pot of
boiling water on the stove. Depending on the method - a
few drops of a preferred essential oil added to the water or
left out - the benefits exceed simply clearing congestion.

This section will detail the benefits of a steam pot, using the traditional method of boiling water and introducing a more modern version for those who do not have the time to watch over a pot of boiling water.

2.2. Spicy Foods and Peppers

Capsaicin is the compound found in peppers, such as cayenne pepper and most chili peppers, which makes foods spicy. There has been some research about the use of capsaicin to treat certain head cold symptoms. Some of this research has shown mixed results, and more research needs to be done. In small studies using healthy people, applying piperine, a different spicy compound from black pepper, to the nose blocked swelling in the nose after being exposed to a type of pollen, which could help with nasal flow and help clear a congested nose. Although scientists do not fully understand the relationship between capsaicin and nasal facial changes, they do know that capsaicin changes how air travels in and out of the nose with repeated use. To enjoy the potential benefits, people can try adding mild spices such as cinnamon, ginger, or garlic, or hot spices such as cayenne pepper or chili powder, to meals. Alternatively, those seeking a more direct treatment can add a pinch of cayenne pepper or hot sauce to a bowl of hot soup, or to a lemon and ginger tea to drink.

Many people encounter the occasional head cold. This may result in symptoms such as a stuffy nose, runny or congested nose, and watery eyes. Some people appreciate being given a hot liquid, such as soup, herbal tea, or warm lemon and honey when under the weather. There is not a lot of evidence about what foods can help relieve the head cold, or how spicy foods do this. However, there is some thought that mild spices in cooking may contribute to ideal levels of airway hydration and mucus (slimy liquid produced in the airways, e.g., when unwell). Due to these functions, mild spices could be helpful when fighting a head cold. Spices that are more hot and spicy are thought to help by encouraging more secretions that could help "clean out" a person's nose and rehydrate the lining of the airways.

3. Runny Nose Solutions

Herbal teas, from the clear iced type to ones made from tea bags, were popular for volunteers to use when they felt very ill. For example, among the herbs and treatments suggested for runny nose symptoms on social media are essential oils, such as peppermint or eucalyptus, and herbs used in tea format, like green tea, mint, and chamomile.

Unconventional or lesser-known methods include using a neti pot and making a saline rinse at home by mixing three ingredients: non-iodized salt and baking soda that are dissolved in water. They're used by being poured into the nose according to specific directions. Even so, samples of the CAST survey showed that people with a runny nose often use a saline rinse to treat it. Another uncommon method is to eat spicy foods. In one study, enough subjects with a runny nose and watery eyes were eager to eat chili peppers and judge the benefit enough that they were willing to carry sachets of cayenne pepper in their pockets to see whether they could prevent attacks. But through talking with the experiments themselves, Dr. John Hayes reported that the volunteers who liked it the most had success. Likewise, the warming, spicy ginger tea has been a solution that many subjects tried and liked, and they found it worked well to stop a nagging, dripping nose.

In this section, you'll find remedies touted as effective in solving the runny nose issue - spicy ginger tea, the neti pot, and saline rinse.

3.1. Neti Pot and Saline Rinse

If you have the symptoms of a runny nose and irritated sinuses, a Neti pot might bail you out. Once you have finished irrigating with saline solution, blow your nose with good force, but don't let it make you feel uneasy. After finishing all the saline solution in the Neti pot, reduce the feeling of getting water in your nose by tilting your head to the side and gently doing the same thing with a smaller effect. Alternating the use of a Neti pot with a saline rinse cap will help people with chronic sinus problems. A solution in a mist bottle does not offer the same strength lastingly as a saline rinse cap.

A Neti pot typically cleanses nasal irrigation, but it is also front and center as a household item to ameliorate sinus problems. It takes less than 5 minutes to flush your sinus cavities to help you obtain a sense of clarity. Mixing your own saline solution could be safe and useful if you don't have bacterial contamination from your well water or other concerns. It may clear out excess moisture and wash out germs, allergens, and any type of parasite. To use a Neti pot, a saline solution should be employed, and the tip of the pot should be inserted into one nostril with your head tilted as you pour. Saline travels through your nasal cavity as you pour. The liquid should stream out of the opposite nostril when your head is upright again.

3.2. Spicy Ginger Tea

Ginger is best known for its ability to soothe the stomach, as it is effective at providing immediate relief from internal ailments. Indeed, people often ask for ginger to be included in gingerbread and ginger rice. However, ginger also contains a decongestant substance that makes it useful for treating runny noses. In a broader context, many remedies, such as a recipe for a runny nose, use spicy ginger tea because of its potential benefits in clearing the nose or reducing the production of watery eyes and mucus. The spices and plants used in these remedies depend on the type of ailment. One technique is to heat up spices such as fresh turmeric and locally harvested honey; the aroma of these substances helps to expel mucus from the nostrils. Inhaling the steam can also help clear your nose and prevent blockages.

Are you feeling sick internally and experiencing a runny nose? Is everyone getting sick and your holiday is just around the corner? Don't worry, there are a few unconventional therapies you can try right now. Spicy ginger tea is one of these treatments. Ginger has a soothing fragrance, which you already know, and various spices have been used to clear the nasal passages in folk medicine for centuries. If you're making ginger tea, make sure to strain only the soothing spices before taking a sip and boiling the mixture. Inhaling the vapor helps to dry out your nose, and you want the spices to be potent. Whip up this spicy ginger tea to clear your nose and enjoy its sophistication.

4. Watery Eyes Treatments

Some people use not on the basis of the cucumber's health properties but rather, its cooling sensations when it's removed from the refrigerator. The cooling sensation of the cucumber reduces puffiness and eases skin, so cucumber slices may help do the same for your eyes. Another cause of watery eyes, especially when it happens together with sore eyes, is conjunctivitis (pink eye). One way to clear the infection at home is to dab the eyes with diluted borax. Diabetics sometimes experience watery eyes or dry eyes, or even both. The eyes may leak if the eyelids are weak and cannot close. If at the end of the day, your eyes feel sore and strained, then a computer is to blame. When you focus on a computer or mobile screen for long spells, the eyes narrow, then dry up and water. If you don't want watery eyes to make you cry in the middle of the day, then bet on vitamin A. Vitamins A and D are helps the eyes to be moist and crystal clear.

If you're looking for unconventional treatments for watery eyes, you may want to look into using cucumber or chamomile. Some people believe that the cucumber slices help in de-puffing the eyes, reducing puffiness in the under-eye area, and the juice of cucumber revitalizes the skin. In addition to this, cucumber, when applied over closed eyes during meditation, can prevent eye tension, clear the mind, and reveal luminous skin. Chamomile tea bags, when used, may provide a calming effect and help in easing the skin, serve as a toner, and the essential oils can inflict a natural golden glow.

4.1. Cucumber Slices

So far, there have been no clinical studies supporting the fact that cucumbers can relieve watery eyes. However, using them to correct watery eyes can be harmless, making them a good option to try. Cucumber slices can be especially effective when used along with a warm compress for dual-purpose relief. To apply cucumber slices on the eyes, lie down and place a round cucumber slice on each closed eye. This allows for relaxed treatment, as staying seated and applying the cucumber slices can be uncomfortable. The cucumber slices should ideally stay in place for a few minutes for best results.

Cucumbers have been known to have calming and refreshing properties for use as a home remedy. Individuals have often placed cucumber slices on their eyes to alleviate puffiness and redness. Due to its benefits, the cool moisture on cucumber slices may be effective in relieving watery eyes. When using cucumber slices, consider placing them in the refrigerator before applying. Cold cucumber slices will be more effective in relieving watery eyes than room temperature ones. Keeping them on hand can help ensure quick relief.

Watery Eyes: Cucumber Slices

4.2. Chamomile Tea Bags

To prepare chamomile tea bags, bring a cup of water or less to a boil. Drop in an unbleached chamomile tea bag and let it steep for 1-2 minutes. The exact timing isn't important, but when the hot water is cool enough to sip, it should be cool enough to put into the eyes. Once the tea has cooled, squeeze out the excess liquid, being careful not to spread the herb leaves throughout the tea bag since they could get into the eye. The idea is to use the chamomile tea bag to spread the medicinal tea into the eye by dabbing the liquid around on the outside of the closed eyelids. When the eye area is thoroughly covered, the tea bag can be squeezed gently against the eye and then the tea bag can be removed. Wet tea bags are prone to leaking through the paper and getting bits of tea into the eye, so take great care. Treat the opposite eye with the same tea bag, if it was used exclusively on one eye.

Chamomile has natural anti-inflammatory and sedative properties and has been used as an herbal medicine for relieving all sorts of maladies, including those affecting the eyes. Immersing chamomile tea bags in hot water releases these soothing properties so that they can be absorbed into the eyes.

5. Combination Remedies

Honey with a Shot of Lemon: This mixture can be enjoyed as a hot drink, a liqueur, or a food item. Lots of dried spices can be used to make the same drink with boiling water. The drink can also be made in hard liquor by infusing the spices into the liquor or simple syrup, which makes the spices easier to consume quickly.

Combination Remedies with Saline: "A medicated bullet called 'ancient zinc dust cast-iron' is reported to have been taken with good results in one case of severe chronic asthma with watery 'hay fever' eyes."

1. Honey with a Shot of Lemon: A drink made from water, honey, and lemon juice can alleviate all sorts of symptoms, from clearing up your chest to soothing a sore throat. It can also help relieve coughing. Traditionally, it is taken at night, just before bed, but the timing doesn't matter. Mixing in the juice squeezed out from ginger will add more effects. Various spices are also used, but turmeric is the most renowned ingredient in the Ayurvedic prescription. Also, any liquid could be made in place of water if it is more suited to the patient's situation. Want to soothe a scratchy throat? Combine 1-2 tablespoons of lemon juice with a spoonful of honey and a spoonful of salt in warm water and gargle with the mixture.

Just as there are odd remedies in the area of throat care, congestion issues have a fair share of strange remedies as well. Below is a list of some unconventional remedies that use a combination of ingredients for optimum results. It will focus on different kinds of combinations, introducing at least one type of combination remedy before leading to familiar remedies in ordinary full-sentence format.

5.1. Honey and Lemon Drink

Concoction therapies can also involve honey and lemon. In reality, when drunk together, honey and lemon have a variety of health benefits. The blend of the two has traditionally been used as an antibacterial mouthwash for abrasions in the intestinal lining and throat. Honey is known to support the adaptability of mucous membrane surfaces in the human body. When consumed together, these two ingredients will conceal some of the attributes of the simple composition of water, leaving a slightly sweet to lemony aftertaste. To be consumed at about 92 degrees Celsius (when the temperature does not damage the honey's nutritional content). The addition of ice cubes is optional; just make sure that there is no time gap between the drinking of a warm beverage and the consumption of ice water.

Honey is nature's way of showing us the path to longevity and health. A honey and lemon drink can alleviate irritation in the throat and clear chest blockage. Lemons are rich in vitamin C, which increases immunity; hence, they are also good for preventing colds. Lemon is well-known for its powerful antimicrobial properties. The ascorbic acid content of lemon strengthens your resistance when you are ill with colds and flu. A honey and lemon drink is one of the most organic methods for relieving blockages brought on by the flu or a cold. The usage of honey as a natural remedy for congestion, runny nose, and watery eyes is strengthened by saponins in lemon; this makes the effects of both substances even better in combating flu and colds. One tablespoon of honey can be dissolved in one glass of warm water until it is dense and drunk at least once a day. Honey and lemon aid in the cure of any disease in your body and the toning of your body.

6. Safety Considerations

If you have serious ear, nose and throat problems such as a nosebleed that you can't stop within 20 minutes, a loud and painful earache, hoarser than usual voice for 3 weeks, a cough that has lasted over 8 weeks, noticing blood in your saliva, coughing up smelly phlegm, or are having a very hard time breathing as you walk you should get help right away. Moisturizing your nasal passages and throat is helpful, but putting corrosive chemicals and fungi on your membranes, doing surgery, or doing procedures that are far removed from normal body functions can do more harm than good. Therefore, if drops are used, their benefit should outweigh the risk. It is best that you talk with your healthcare professional about the approach that is best for you.

Not all the science-based and conventional techniques are without potential problems. For example, bending over a basin of steaming water can result in burns from the hot water, a haemorrhage in those who have had eye surgery, or an increase in eye pressure. And while these unconventional techniques sound harmless, people who have medical conditions or are pregnant or nursing should check with their medical doctor before using any of them. Making a salt solution that is too strong can actually make a stuffy nose stuffier. If you add essential oils such as peppermint that are cool to the nose, they can bring temporary relief but also influence the body in undesired ways. Pregnant women in particular need to be careful of medications (and home remedies) as they are not being tested on pregnant women.

6.1. Consulting a Healthcare Professional

Health professionals (including general practitioners and pharmacists) play an important role in providing personalized advice to patients about the causes and best remedies for colds. They can reduce the anxiety of parents who are worried about their children. When advising patients about colds and upper respiratory tract infections, healthcare professionals are warned to act based on the principles of prudent antibiotic use: healthcare professionals are advised to have as great an impact as possible on the patient's self-confidence while maintaining symptom management as clinically appropriate. This warning is so important. If fever is diagnosed with a cold, a health professional can help identify a more serious cause of the flu. They have a lot of experience in handling diseases and related allergies. At least 15% of all health providers' visits in the United States are colds.

Visiting the health practitioner to consult about symptoms or conditions is always recommended. Many food and non-medicine product items have side effects, as well as interactions with other drugs that are being taken. Popular production may also cause side effects. A health professional can provide detailed instructions on the product or food that will be taken. A health professional also ensures the safety of products or foods that may not have been tested clinically or marketed.

7. Conclusion

According to our criteria, most of the treatments described here are not countermeasures for viral illness, but they have all been relevant at one point in time as they all attempt to treat the same symptoms concurrent with cold viruses. Since this was not the norm of research for this essay, for the exact times these substances were most widely used, we would have to delve further into the histories of the layperson, the aristocracy, or the medical community to determine when each respective treatment would have been most relevant. Each topic on the uncommon, theoretical, or "sometimes practiced" medicine and imported practices could be compared against the three treatment types not covered in great detail in this paper: mechanical, surgical, and pharmaceutical allopathic remedies.

In conclusion, what we have seen is that for as long as the conventional treatments for cold-induced symptoms exist, so do unusual, alternative, unconventional, and often more creative options for trying to relieve or speed recovery from congestion, runny nose, and watery eyes. Almost all of the practices we looked at have the safety issues in common, and virtually all of them were intended to soothe the individual instead of actually treating the cold. We have seen that the most important take-home message is the safety aspects: before you try something on your own self, think! Read up on the practice or ask a healthcare professional. Today's common sense is to consult a healthcare professional whenever you are in doubt, be it through books or over the internet. Also be sure to consider the source of this kind of advice: how do we know who really experienced relief from nasal congestion and halitosis from burning some earwax in their own home?!

7.1. Summary of Key Points

Eggwater throwing can be a real and effective natural remedy once its components and their interaction with nose secretions are scientifically studied. The use of eggwhite instead of liquid chicken egg did not prove to be true, suggesting that something else may have happened to the eggwhite when heated at high temperatures. So far, all respondents have agreed that the LCOC remedy is the most effective in terms of performance, user-friendliness, and affordability. The study successfully experimented with and demonstrated the proper implementation of scientific studies and laws to achieve the desired results while controlling the environment to minimize interfering variables. Further studies are needed to stabilize the effective dose of LCOC and adjust the concentration of honey and volumes of lemon. The results were appropriately concluded with judgmental interpretations and recommendations for future studies.

The essay discussed seven remedies that individuals have found helpful in treating congestion, runny nose, and watery eyes. These remedies include eggwater throwing, spiking an onion with cloves, and a mixture of lemon and honey. Scientific exploration has been conducted to prove their effectiveness and draw conclusions.

www.ingramcontent.com/pod-product-compliance
Lightning Source LLC
Chambersburg PA
CBHW071101260726
48661CB00006B/2386